KT-367-509

Overcoming Common Problems Series

Overcoming Common Problems Series

Dr Dawn's Guide to Sexual Health

Dr Dawn Harper is a GP based in Gloucestershire, working at an NHS surgery in Stroud. She has been working as a media doctor for nearly ten years. Dawn is best known as one of the presenters on Channel 4's award-winning programme *Embarrassing Bodies*, which has run for seven series and last year celebrated its hundredth episode. Spin-offs have included *Embarrassing Fat Bodies*, *Embarrassing Teen Bodies* and *Embarrassing Bodies: Live from the clinic*.

Dawn is the presenter of Channel 4's series *Born Naughty?*, one of the doctors on ITV1's *This Morning* and the resident GP on the health hour on LBC radio. She writes for a variety of publications, including *Healthspan*, *Healthy Food Guide* and *NetDoctor*. Her first book, *Dr Dawn's Health Check*, was published by Mitchell Beazley. *Dr Dawn's Guide to Sexual Health* is one of five Dr Dawn Guides published by Sheldon Press in 2016. Dawn qualified at London University in 1987. When not working, she is a keen cyclist and an enthusiastic supporter of children's charities. Her website is at <www.drdawn.com>. Follow her on Twitter @drdawnharper.

Overcoming Common Problems Series

Selected titles

A full list of titles is available from Sheldon Press,
36 Causton Street, London SW1P 4ST and on our website at
www.sheldonpress.co.uk

Overcoming Common Problems

Dr Dawn's Guide to Sexual Health

DR DAWN HARPER

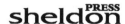
sheldon **PRESS**

First published in Great Britain in 2016

Sheldon Press
36 Causton Street
London SW1P 4ST
www.sheldonpress.co.uk

British Library Cataloguing-in-Publication Data
A catalogue record for this book is available from the British Library

ISBN 978–1–84709–391–2
eBook ISBN 978–1–84709–396–7

Typeset by Fakenham Photosetting Ltd, Fakenham, Norfolk
Typeset by Fakenham Prepress Solutions, Fakenham, Norfolk NR21 8NN
Subsequently digitally reprinted in Great Britain

eBook by Fakenham Prepress Solutions, Fakenham, Norfolk NR21 8NN

Produced on paper from sustainable forests

Contents

Note to the reader

This is not a medical book and is not intended to replace advice from your doctor. Consult your pharmacist or doctor if you believe you have any of the symptoms described, and if you think you might need medical help.

1

The female reproductive system – anatomy and function

I thought I would start by defining what we mean by the female reproductive system. I remember doing some filming on what is normal and what is not when it comes to your vulva and in a group of 20 women there was a lot of confusion about what your vulva is and indeed what you call it! The vulva is the external genitalia: the labia majora and minora, the clitoris and the opening to the vagina. We are undoubtedly better at talking more openly today than we used to be but there is still a degree of taboo about all things sexual, so let's start with a look at what comprises the female genitals, both internal and external (Figure 1).

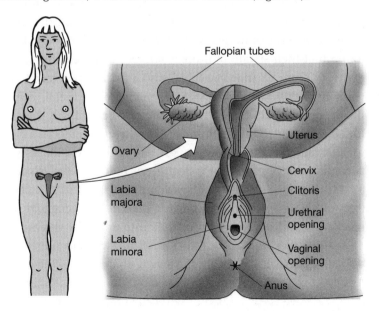

Figure 1 The female genitalia

1

The external genital organs

- **The labia majora** are the large fleshy lips covered with skin and, after puberty, with pubic hair. The skin contains sweat and oil secreting glands.

- **The labia minora**, or 'small lips', lie just inside the labia majora and surround the entrance to the vagina. They are barely visible externally in pre-pubertal girls but grow during puberty and vary significantly in size. In recent years I have seen increasing numbers of young women concerned that their labia minora are larger than they should be and asking for surgical correction. In most cases they are anatomically completely normal and I simply have to reassure of them of that fact. My guess is there are a number of reasons for their concerns. Young women today tend to remove most or all of their pubic hair, which of course makes the labia look more prominent. Young women also tend to wear thong underwear, which may predispose them to some chafing. In most instances I try not to refer for surgery as it is generally a bigger procedure than most women realize and, we mustn't forget, the labia minora have a function and that is to channel the flow of urine. I have met several women who have found that their stream of urine is poorly controlled after labioplasty (surgery to trim the labia) and subsequently regret the decision.

- **Bartholin's glands** These are a pair of pea-sized glands that are found either side of the entrance to the vagina and secrete fluid to lubricate the vagina during sex. Sometimes the ducts can become blocked, causing a collection of fluid in what is called a Bartholin's cyst. If the glands become infected, this is called a Bartholin's abscess. This can be very painful and generally will need antibiotics and often an operation to drain the abscess.

- **The clitoris** is found at the junction of the two labia minora, at the top. It varies in size and is the female equivalent of the penis. As such it is highly sensitive and can swell during sexual stimulation. It is covered by a hood of skin called the prepuce.

The internal genital organs

These include:

- **The vagina** This is the elastic, muscular canal that runs from the labia minora on the outside to the neck of the womb, or cervix, on the inside. It is lined by a delicate mucosa that has glands to produce fluid to keep the vagina lubricated and nerve endings to provide sensation. There are millions of bacteria that keep our vaginas clean and in balance. If these bacteria get out of kilter you may notice a change in the amount, odour or colour of your normal vaginal discharge. It is important not to over wash your vagina. It is effectively a self-cleaning organ so simple water should be enough. Try to avoid douching, which may wash out some of the healthy bacteria, or perfumed products, which alter the naturally acidic pH of the vagina, resulting in an overgrowth of some bacteria. The vagina accepts the penis during intercourse and acts as a channel for the flow of blood during menstruation or for a baby during a vaginal delivery.
- **The hymen** is the delicate membrane at the opening of the vagina. It is stretched during intercourse but can also be stretched at other times so cannot be relied on as a sign of virginity.
- **The uterus (womb)** The non-pregnant uterus is about the size and shape of a small pear, but it can expand to accommodate a growing foetus.
- **The cervix** This is the neck of the womb. It can be felt, with a finger, at the top of your vagina. Your cervix should feel like the tip of your nose and you may notice a dimple in the middle. This is the cervical os – the opening in the cervix that leads to the womb. This opens slightly to allow menstrual blood to leave the uterus and dilates significantly during labour.
- **The fallopian tubes** are two narrow tubes that attach to the upper part of the uterus. At the other end they fan out to form what are called fimbriae so that they can catch eggs released from the ovaries. The eggs are passed along the fallopian tubes. If an

egg meets a sperm along its way the egg is then fertilized along the fallopian tube and implanted into the womb lining. If the egg is not fertilized it will continue to make its way along the tube and will be expelled, along with the uterine lining, which is what you notice as a period.

- **The ovaries** are small, almond-shaped and -sized organs that produce eggs and hormones. Women are born with a fixed number of eggs which they will release at a rate of about one a month throughout their menstruating life. Men, on the other hand, continue to produce new sperm throughout most of their adult lives. On average, assuming both ovaries are healthy, women produce half their eggs from the left ovary and half from the right but they are not necessarily produced in a strictly alternating pattern.

Sexual function

I hesitate to use the word 'normal' here because, of course, every woman's experience of sexual function is very personal and can vary from day to day and throughout life. What is 'normal' and fulfilling for one woman may not be for the next, but bear with me while I try to talk through what I see as the four stages of female sexual function.

Sexual desire or libido

Few women would argue that the female libido is complex. I have a lovely friend who lectures regularly on the subject and uses a couple of slides to illustrate her talk. The female libido she likens to a remote control. There are 20 or 30 buttons with labels for everything from 'time of the month', 'work stress', 'kids' homework' and 'how tidy is the house?'. She always gets a laugh and goes on to say not only is the remote very complex but that in order for the right channel to be selected, the buttons need to be pressed in a particular order! She of course gets a further laugh when she shows the male remote, which simply reads 'beer' and 'sex'! To be fair to men I am, of course, over simplifying things and we will discuss male sexual function in the next chapter.

Arousal

The initial response to sexual stimulation is vascular dilation, allowing engorgement of the genital tissues followed by changes in the nerves and muscles, enabling the vagina to balloon and the clitoris to retract slightly.

Orgasm

The muscles around the vagina contract and the woman feels a sensation of climax.

Resolution

During this phase all the changes described above gradually reverse.

Does the G spot exist?

The existence of the G spot, or Gräfenberg spot, has caused something of a debate over the years. It is supposed to be an area on the inside of the front wall of the vagina, about 5 cm inside, which is highly sensitive and thought to be responsible for orgasm during penetration. Modern imaging techniques have allowed scientists to study the vagina during sexual stimulation and intercourse. They have identified that the vagina plays a very active role in sexual arousal and during sex. There also seems to be a region between the clitoris, urethra and vagina that, if stimulated, could lead to orgasm during penetration, although most women tell me that they reach orgasm during clitoral stimulation rather than during penetration.

2

The male reproductive system – anatomy and function

Unlike the female reproductive system, nearly all the male genitalia are seen outside of the body (Figure 2).

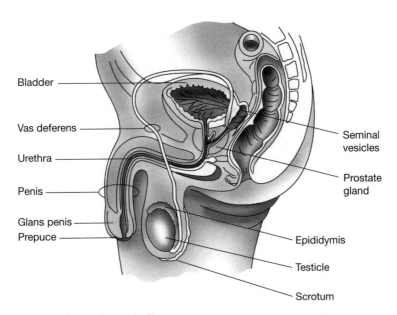

Figure 2 The male genitalia

- **The penis** This is the male organ through which men urinate and which is used during sexual intercourse. It has three parts – the root, which is the base of the penis attached to the rest of the body; the shaft, which is the main part consisting of three circular chambers; and the glans, or head, of the penis. This, just like the female clitoris, has lots of sensitive nerve endings. In about one in five men, you may notice thin white spots around the base of the glans. These are called pearly penile papules. They get their name because they can look like a string of pearls. They are completely benign and you shouldn't try to pick at them to remove them as you risk them becoming infected and then leaving a scar. The glans is loosely covered with a layer of skin called the foreskin, which should be able to be retracted. It can be removed in the procedure known as a circumcision. Throughout the length of the penis runs the urethra, which carries urine from the bladder to the outside world. During intercourse, the penis becomes erect, which squeezes the urethra so that only semen is produced during ejaculation.

- **The scrotum** This is the loose bag of skin that houses the testicles. It hangs behind and below the penis and one side tends to hang lower than the other. The skin is often slightly more pigmented than the surrounding skin and covered in pubic hair after puberty. It also contains many oil secreting glands and sweat glands. I often see men concerned about small white spots in the skin of the scrotum, which are very common and are usually simply benign cysts. On the outside of the scrotum, in the midline, you will notice a ridge of skin called the raphe which attaches inside to a septum, which separates the two testicles. The main function of the scrotum is to hold the testicles in place outside of the body where they can remain cool, which is good for the production of healthy sperm. In warm conditions the muscular lining of the scrotal sack stretches to allow the testes to hang lower and stay cooler, while in cold conditions the muscle may contract to bring the testes closer to the warm body.

- **The testicles** Most men have two testicles and they are about 4–5 cm long and 2–3 cm in diameter, weighing about 25 grams each. In the foetus, the testicles develop inside the abdomen and only descend into the scrotal sac towards the end of pregnancy. In about two in every hundred male births, one or both testicles have failed to descend, but this usually corrects itself by the time the child is three months old. Doctors routinely check that testicles are descended though and will want to follow up because undescended testicles stay warmer than they should and this can have an effect on future fertility, as well as having a slight increased risk of testicular cancer. There is a reflex which retracts the testicle back into the abdomen and, even into adult life, if you tickle the inner upper thigh the testicles will retract. This is not a problem as the risks only apply to testicles that stay in the abdominal cavity. Inside, the testicles are divided into hundreds of tiny lobes containing cells, which produce sperm. Men are not born with sperm. They produce sperm on a daily basis from puberty.
- **The epididymis** This is a long tube at the back of the testicle. It stores freshly made sperm from the testicles and allows them to mature.
- **The vas deferens** This is the muscular tube that carries sperm from the epididymis to the urethra ready for ejaculation. It is this tube that we cut during a vasectomy.
- **Seminal vesicles** These are found at the end of the vas deferens near the base of the bladder and they are responsible for producing a sugar-rich fluid. This provides a source of energy for sperm, which need to swim hard to reach an egg. Contrary to popular belief most of a man's ejaculate is actually this seminal fluid and not sperm, which is why it is perfectly possible to have what appears to be normal ejaculate but not be fertile.
- **The prostate gland** is a walnut-shaped gland that lies at the base of the bladder surrounding the urethra. It also produces fluid to help nourish the sperm.
- **The bulbourethral glands (Cowper's glands)** These are tiny

pea-sized glands that lie at the base of the prostate and they produce fluid to lubricate the urethra but also to neutralize any residual drops of urine, which will be slightly acidic.

How does an erection occur?

As mentioned above, the penis has three circular chambers. These are made up of spongy tissue that is full of blood vessels. When a man is sexually aroused, the brain sends messages to the blood vessels in the penis allowing them to dilate. At the same time a ring of muscle at the base of the penis tightens so that blood can flow in but not out. This makes the penis engorged with blood and stiff, which is what we recognize as an erection. When the state of sexual arousal resolves, the ring of muscle relaxes again, allowing the blood to flow out, and the penis reverts to its flaccid state.

Penises come in all shapes and sizes, just like hands, feet and noses. You may have heard the terms 'growers' and 'showers' and this refers to the fact that whatever the size of the penis when it is flaccid, the average erect penis is usually very similar in size measuring 14–16 cm in length with a girth of 12–13 cm. The length measurement is taken from the base of the penis, on the side of the tummy, to the tip.

Men are often concerned about the size of their penis, believing that it is not big enough. One possible explanation for this is that when a man looks down on his penis it may look smaller than when viewed from the front or the side. So, standing in a urinal or in a shower, it is possible to think that the men around you are larger than you. To see your penis the way others do you should look at it front on in a full-length mirror.

It is normal to have several erections during the day and night and men will often wake in the morning with an erection. The frequency of erections varies from man to man and tends to become less frequent with age, so young men may have 10–20 erections a day but this tends to become less frequent with age.

How does ejaculation occur?

Ejaculation is the release of sperm and seminal fluid at the point of orgasm. It occurs when a man reaches the climax of sexual excitement and the nerve endings in the penis send messages to the brain, which then sends messages back to the penis leading to ejaculation. Ejaculation occurs in two phases. In the first phase, the seminal vesicles and the vas deferens squeeze seminal fluid and sperm towards the back of the urethra. This triggers receptors in the back of the urethra, which causes the muscles at the base of the penis to contract strongly. This is the second phase. The contractions occur every 0.8 of a second forcing the semen out of the tip of the penis. Contrary to popular belief, you don't need an erection to achieve ejaculation.

What is semen?

Semen is made up of sperm and secretions from the seminal vesicles, prostate and other glands found in the genital tract. It is slightly alkaline (pH 7.2–7.8) and usually tastes salty because, like tears and sweat, it does contain some salt. Normally, it is clear or white in colour and when first produced it tends to be thick and slightly sticky, becoming more watery over time. If it has a yellow tinge this may suggest infection and if it is pink or brown it could mean there is blood in it. Blood in the semen (haematospermia) isn't necessarily serious – in fact, the most common cause for blood in the semen is overzealous masturbation or sexual intercourse, but if there is any possibility of infection it should be checked out by a doctor.

How quickly should I be able to achieve an erection after orgasm?

After ejaculation a man goes into what is called the refractory period. This is, in effect, a type of recovery when he won't think about sex and is not sexually aroused. The time of the refractory period is not linked to potency or testosterone levels and can vary hugely in different men. Age seems to play a significant role, so a man in his teens or early twenties may be able to achieve another erection within minutes of ejaculation while a man in his seventies may spend 24 hours or longer in the refractory period.

3

Female sexual development

We are all individuals and when we start and end puberty will vary from woman to woman, but the way we develop physically tends to follow a pattern. This pattern was first described by Professor James Tanner who was an expert in child development, and we now use what we call the Tanner stages to describe normal puberty.

Tanner stage 1

This is the pre-pubertal body, namely the way a girl looks before puberty begins.

Tanner stage 2

This usually occurs around the age of 11. Initially breast buds develop. These are small swellings behind the nipple. They may be quite tender and it is common for them to develop unevenly to begin with. Sometimes a girl may have a breast bud on one side and nothing on the other for several months. The pigmented area around the nipple, the areola, may begin to swell and fine pubic hair will begin to grow, usually starting along the labia majora, the outer lips. The womb also begins to grow at this time but you will be unaware of that. There is also a growth spurt and it is normal to grow 7–8 cm in a year.

Tanner stage 3

This usually occurs after the age of 12. The breasts continue to develop and this may be about the time you buy your first bra. Pubic hair becomes thicker and curlier and you will start to grow armpit hair. You may notice your hair feels greasier and you may develop spots on your skin. You will grow about 8 cm in a year.

Tanner stage 4

This usually occurs around 13. Breasts continue to develop into a more adult shape and the nipple and areola become prominent above the level of the breast tissue. Pubic hair looks more like adult pubic hair but is still confined to the mons pubis – the mound of fatty tissue that lies over the pubic bone – and does not spread to the inner thighs. At this time, 90 per cent of girls will start their periods. It is normal for the first few periods to be erratic and pain free, but over the next 6–12 months they should become more regular and you may notice they become heavier and more painful. You will still be growing but the rate will slow to around 7 cm a year.

Tanner stage 5

This occurs around the age of 14. Breasts take on a more adult shape and pubic hair spreads to the inner thighs. You will continue to grow another 5–7.5 cm over the two years after your periods start and this will be your adult height.

Throughout puberty, as your hormones kick in, it is normal to be on a bit of an emotional rollercoaster. You may feel tearful at times and have unexpected mood swings but these should disappear as your hormones settle.

4

Male sexual development

Just like girls, boys will vary as to when they start puberty but they also follow a pattern which is described, in the same way, in five Tanner stages.

Tanner stage 1

This is the pre-pubertal stage.

Tanner stage 2

This usually starts around 12 (a year later than girls). The skin of the scrotum will become thinner and redder. The testicles will start to increase in size, and fine pubic hair will begin to appear around the base of the penis.

Tanner stage 3

This occurs after 13. The testicles continue to grow and the penis begins to grow longer. Pubic hair becomes thicker and curlier and spreads to the skin above the base of the penis. About one in three boys will notice some swelling of their breast tissue but this will settle over time. It is around this time that you may notice that you have ejaculated in your sleep. This is called a 'wet dream'. It is around now that the voice starts to break, which means you may notice that the pitch and tone of your voice may suddenly alter for periods of time. Boys tend to become more muscular around this time and will grow at around 7–8 cm a year.

Tanner stage 4

This occurs around the age of 14. The penis and testicles continue to grow and the scrotal skin becomes darker. Pubic hair looks more like adult hair but it doesn't spread to the inner thighs. Armpit hair begins to grow and the voice deepens permanently. Hair may appear more greasy and you may develop spots.

Tanner stage 5

This usually occurs at about 15. Pubic hair spreads to the inner thighs and the penis, scrotum and testicles look more like an adult's. You will start to grow facial hair and may need to begin shaving. The growth spurt will slow down but you will continue to grow and develop until about the age of 18.

Just like girls, hormonal changes in puberty may mean you experience mood swings and may feel angry at times.

5

Menstrual problems

The average age to start periods in the UK is 13. This is younger than a century ago and is probably down to improved nutrition and increasing weight. There is a critical weight at which our hormones kick in and, in fact, at which they shut down, which is why very thin athletes and anorexic girls often stop having periods altogether. But starting your periods anywhere between 8 and 16 is normal – girls who start their periods before the age of 8 should be investigated, as should those who are yet to see their first period after the age of 16.

What is a normal cycle?

We talk of a normal menstrual cycle as being 28 days with ovulation occurring in the middle but anything from 21 days to 35 is considered within normal limits. If you are trying to predict ovulation, it is important to remember that ovulation occurs 14 days *before* the first day of a period, not 14 days *after* a period. Of course, in the context of a 28 day cycle these are one and the same but, if you have a regular, 21 day cycle for example, your fertile time (when you ovulate) will be 14 days before your period which is just 7 days after day 1 of your previous period (day 1 being the first day of bleeding). Worth bearing in mind if you are timing sex to avoid your fertile time or are trying to conceive!

As your period starts, a gland in your brain called the pituitary gland is already producing a hormone, called follicle stimulating hormone (FSH), which as its name suggests stimulates the development of follicles in your ovary. As a follicle matures it produces oestrogen and as oestrogen levels rise, messages are fed back to the brain to stop producing FSH. Once oestrogen levels are high enough, the pituitary produces a second hormone, luteinizing hormone (LH). This surge of LH is what triggers ovulation which occurs within about 36 hours. The egg is released from the ovary and travels along the fallopian tube to the womb where the lining has thickened ready to nurture a fertilized egg and develop a pregnancy. If pregnancy does not occur, that thickened lining is shed and this is what we recognize as a period. And then the cycle starts all over again.

What is normal blood loss?

All women vary and each individual will notice differences in their periods from time to time. Average blood loss has been calculated by scientists though and is thought to be around 40 ml per period. That is just eight teaspoons over the average five or six days that a woman bleeds. I find that women are often surprised by how little that is. It feels a lot more, doesn't it, but you only have to see a child with a nose bleed to see that a small amount of blood can go a long way!

What is heavy menstrual bleeding?

Heavy periods or menorrhagia (coming from the Greek *men*, meaning month, and *rhegynai*, to rush out) are one of the most common complaints doctors hear about periods. Strictly speaking the definition of menorrhagia is a blood loss of more than 16 teaspoons (80 ml). If left untreated this sort of blood loss will almost certainly lead to anaemia so needs to be treated. But who measures their menstrual loss? Those using a moon cup to collect menstrual blood rather than pads or tampons may have a more accurate idea but, as far as I am concerned, if you feel your periods are heavy and they are interfering with your day-to-day life then we need to help you.

And, of course, what is acceptable to one woman will be totally unacceptable to another for lots of different reasons. It may be related to what you are used to, or to your mother's and sister's experiences. Some women are more robust than others and, of course, what you have to do in your day will have an influence too. If you work from home and don't have to go out, heavy periods are much less likely to cause you problems than if you are having to travel long distances or spend hours in meetings unable to get to a loo. However, passing clots and flooding are generally accepted as heavy periods and are not something you have to put up with.

What will my doctor do if I complain of heavy periods?

Your GP will want to take a detailed history from you, so before you make the appointment try to make a note of how long this has been a problem, how many days you bleed for and how frequently, and if you can give your doctor an idea of how frequently you are changing pads or tampons that will be helpful too. If it is normal for you to need to use pads and tampons together you are almost certainly putting up with something you shouldn't be!

Your GP will want to examine you to look at the cervix to check for polyps, which can cause abnormal bleeding, and to do an internal examination to check the size of the uterus. If the uterus is enlarged, your doctor will arrange an ultrasound. By far the most common cause of an enlarged uterus (apart from pregnancy when of course your periods will have stopped!) is fibroids. Fibroids are very common – around half of all women over 50 years old will have fibroids. They often don't cause any trouble at all and tend to shrink after the menopause but if they do cause problems, they are most likely to lead to heavy menstrual bleeding. Often we don't find a specific cause, in which case doctors refer to this as dysfunctional uterine bleeding.

Your doctor will also arrange a blood test to check your heavy bleeding hasn't left you anaemic and if he or she is concerned that you have a problem with your thyroid (which can be linked to heavy periods), or a more generalized problem with easy bleeding, he or she may check those blood tests too.

What treatments are available for heavy periods?

The first line of treatment is usually something called an intra-uterine system, which is like a contraceptive coil but which secretes tiny amounts of hormone into the lining of the womb to reduce blood flow. It is very effective and can be fitted by your GP or family planning clinic. The amount of hormone that is released into your system is the same as taking two mini pills a week.

If this is not suitable for you, your doctor may suggest some anti-inflammatory type pills on prescription that can reduce blood flow by between 25 and 50 per cent. They are only taken around the time of bleeding and are non-hormonal. Alternatively, you could try the combined contraceptive pill, which reduces blood flow by around a half.

If none of these measures work, you may be referred for an endometrial ablation. This is a day case procedure done under anaesthetic where the lining of the womb is removed but the womb itself is left in place. It is so effective that the number of hysterecto-mies that are performed each year in the UK has fallen dramatically since this technique was developed.

Other options are to block the artery supplying the womb, a pro-cedure known as uterine artery embolization, to remove the muscle of the womb (myomectomy) or, as a last resort, to perform a full hysterectomy and remove the entire womb.

In other words, there are lots of different treatment options open to you. I have met too many women who have put up with heavy periods for too long because they thought it was a hysterectomy or nothing and they didn't want such a major operation. So if you are struggling don't put up with it any more – make that appointment!

Painful periods (dysmenorrhoea)

Most of us will get some pain with our periods but around one in ten women suffer with so much pain that their periods prevent them getting on with their day-to-day life. Severe pain with periods is more common in younger women and the good news is that things often improve as we get older. There isn't usually any specific cause but if painful periods start in your 30s or 40s then it could be linked to a problem in the pelvis. This is called secondary dysmenorrhoea. Let's deal with the far more common form, primary dysmenorrhoea, first.

Primary dysmenorrhoea

We don't really know why this affects some women and not others. There are a couple of theories though – one is that the chemicals called prostaglandins that build up in the lining of the womb and help it to contract and shed build up in higher concentrations in some women; another is that some women are simply more sensitive to their effect. Period pain, just like labour pain, can be felt in the lower tummy, in the thighs and/or lower back. It usually start a day or so before the bleeding begins and can last for a few days.

What can my doctor do?

Your GP will listen to your story and unless there are specific things that make him or her suspect a secondary cause (see Secondary dysmenorrhoea) probably won't need to examine you. There are various things your doctor may advise depending on the severity of your symptoms. Simple measures like holding a hot water bottle against your tummy or taking paracetamol may suffice for relatively mild symptoms, but women struggling with more severe symptoms may need to take anti-inflammatory drugs. Some, like ibuprofen, you can buy over the counter at the pharmacy but others will need a prescription from your GP.

Taking the combined contraceptive pill tends to lighten periods and make them less painful and there are other progestogen contraceptives that may help if you can't take oestrogen. The intrauterine system used to lighten (or, in many women, stop) periods is another option.

I am often asked about more natural remedies such as herbal or dietary supplements. The jury is out on this – there is no good evidence that they are effective, so my feeling is that more work needs to be done to assess their role before we recommend them.

Secondary dysmenorrhoea

Secondary dysmenorrhoea is when periods suddenly become painful having not been a problem before. It is normal for the first few periods that a girl has to be painless and then as the cycles regulate to become more painful, but if an older woman starts having problems this is called secondary dysmenorrhoea. If the pain is associated with a change in bleeding pattern, bleeding between periods, a vaginal discharge or pain during sex, your GP will want to investigate further with a pelvic examination and possibly other tests, such as an ultrasound of your womb or a examination with a telescope, called a laparoscope, looking around the outside of your womb through a small cut near your tummy button, or a hysteroscope looking inside the womb through your cervix. From there, the treatment will depend on what the tests reveal.

Absent periods (amenorrhoea)

Just like dysmenorrhoea, amenorrhoea can be primary (periods never start) or secondary (periods were normal but have now stopped).

What causes primary amenorrhoea?

The average age to start periods in the UK is 13 but we are all different and some girls will start sooner and others later. If periods haven't started by the age of 16, your doctor may want to do some tests to look into possible causes. Some girls may have been born without a womb, which, of course, is only obvious when periods don't start and an ultrasound confirms its absence. It is also possible to be born with a womb but no passage to the outside. In this case girls may notice period-type pains each month but no bleeding. If periods never start and there are no other signs of puberty such as breast development and pubic hair then there could be a hormonal problem, or this could be caused by some rare syndrome, so your GP will want to arrange some tests.

What causes secondary amenorrhoea?

By far and away the most common cause of secondary amenorrhoea is pregnancy and since no form of contraception is 100 per cent effective, if your periods suddenly stop, a pregnancy test should be your first port of call! The second is probably the menopause and while the average age for the menopause in the UK is 50–2, it is possible to go through the change much earlier. A menopause before 40 is described as a premature menopause and I have met women in their twenties who are going through 'the change'. Your GP will be able to test for this with blood tests.

Other causes include breast feeding and some forms of progesterone-only contraception such as the injection, the implant and the intra-uterine system. It is also relatively common to find that there is a delay in starting periods after stopping the combined contraceptive pill. Periods usually resume within 6 months though, and if they don't, other possibilities should be checked out. Significant weight loss will also stop periods as nature considers very thin women to be unable to carry a healthy pregnancy so shuts down your hormones, which is why anorexic girls and some very thin athletes stop their periods. Polycystic ovaries are another common cause.

There are other rare causes such as severe narrowing of the neck of the womb, and diseases affecting the pituitary gland in the brain that produces the hormones to drive the ovaries.

What about abnormal menstrual bleeding?

Bleeding that occurs after sex (post-coital bleeding), between periods (inter-menstrual bleeding) and bleeding after a woman has gone through the menopause (post-menopausal bleeding) should always be reported to your doctor.

Post-coital bleeding (PCB)

The most common cause of this is an erosion on the cervix. These are particularly common in women taking the combined contraceptive pill and don't usually cause any problems but, if they do, bleeding after sex is a frequent one. Your doctor will be able to see if you have an erosion with a speculum examination, just like when you have a smear. If the problem persists, your cervix can be painted with a special paint to dry up the erosion. You may need more than one treatment. Polyps in the cervical canal or in the womb can also cause post-coital bleeding. Gynaecological cancers such as cancer of the vagina, cervix or womb can also cause these symptoms, which is why it is so important not to ignore them.

Inter-menstrual bleeding (IMB)

In a very small number of women bleeding mid cycle is just a sign of ovulation, but this really is only one or two in every hundred and far more commonly IMB is down to missed contraceptive pills or a sexually transmitted infection. In fact, unless there is an obvious cause such as missed pills, I assume that IMB is due to chlamydia or gonorrhoea until proved otherwise and it is important that these infections are tested for. Things like fibroids and gynaecological cancers can also cause IMB but if there is any suggestion that this is the case, your GP will arrange the necessary tests.

Post-menopausal bleeding (PMB)

Post-menopausal bleeding is defined as bleeding that occurs 12 or more months after the menopause and it should always be looked into. Most cases will not be anything to be worry about but, just like IMB being chlamydia until proved otherwise, uterine cancer must always be excluded in any woman with PMB. Your GP will test for this with an ultrasound test to check out the thickness of the uterine lining and an endometrial biopsy. This can be done by your doctor and involves a tiny instrument being inserted through the cervix to take a sample of cells from the womb lining for analysis under a microscope. I have done literally hundreds of these and had very few positive results, but it is always better to be safe than sorry.

Toxic shock syndrome (TSS)

Toxic shock syndrome is one of those conditions that just about every menstruating woman has heard of and is terrified of, but in fact in all my years of practice I have only ever seen one case. In contrast, I have removed hundreds of forgotten tampons which have been left for days and sometimes even weeks. That said, current recommendations are that tampons should not be left in place for more than eight hours. Thankfully, TSS is rare and, due to developments in tampon manufacture, is becoming more so, but it is a life-threatening condition so one we must consider. TSS presents with a high fever and there may be an associated red rash all over the body. It can cause sickness and diarrhoea and muscle aches. These symptoms can easily be put down to food poisoning or the like so always just think about whether a tampon could have been left inside, because if TSS is left undiagnosed, a patient can rapidly deteriorate, becoming confused and developing kidney and liver failure. High dose antibiotics given promptly will treat the condition but delay could be fatal: 5–15 per cent of people developing TSS will not survive.

6

Contraception

One in four women in the UK use the combined oral contraceptive pill (often referred to as 'the pill') for contraception. It is a very effective form of contraception but no form of contraception is 100 per cent effective. The combined pill is one of the safest as long as it is used properly. If pills are missed, then it becomes far less effective. We know that one in four children in the UK are not planned. That doesn't necessarily mean they are not wanted but many may be a result of late or missed pills. If you are absolutely certain you don't want to fall pregnant at the moment and, hand on heart, your schedule is a little hectic and taking a pill at the same time every day is going to be a challenge, then the 'pill' may not be right for you at the moment. There are lots of options out there so let's look at them.

Pills and patches

The combined oral contraceptive pill

As I have said, one of the most commonly used forms of contraception is the combined oral contraceptive pill (COCP). As its name implies it is a combination of oestrogen and progesterone. It needs to be taken at the same time every day, although you do have a 12 hour window. If taken regularly, it is extremely effective. In fact if a thousand women take it absolutely by the book, only three would become pregnant in a year. But that number could rise to 90 if it is taken less reliably. It works mainly by preventing you from ovulating, but it also has an action on cervical mucus, making it thicker and therefore more difficult for sperm to penetrate and it makes the lining of the womb thinner. This means it is more difficult for an egg to implant, but also explains why many women notice they have lighter, less painful periods while on the combined pill.

It is best to start the pill on the first day of your period and then you are protected straight away, but it can be started anywhere in your cycle as long as you are sure you are not pregnant. If it is after day five (or earlier if you have a short cycle of 23 days or less), then you will need to use condoms as well for the first seven days.

What are the side effects and risks of taking the pill?

When you first take the pill you may notice some side effects including headaches, bloating, breast tenderness and nausea. Women worry about putting on weight on the COCP and it is not uncommon to put on a few pounds but research has shown this is not a side effect of the pill itself. It is more likely to be due to the fact that when you are in a relationship you may be eating and drinking more and it may be a time in your life when you are doing less formal exercise. There are some more serious side effects to consider though. The pill can cause a rise in blood pressure. There is a very small increased risk of blood clots and this is mostly in women with a family history of blood clots, smokers, the very inactive or the very overweight. There is also a very small increased risk of breast and cervical cancer in long-term users.

Who shouldn't take the pill?

You should not take the combined pill if you:

- are significantly obese (body mass index greater than 35);
- smoke and are over 35;
- have high blood pressure;
- have established vascular disease or diabetic complications;
- have a history of blood clots;
- have migraine with aura;
- have blood disorders that make you more prone to clotting;
- are breastfeeding;
- have breast or liver cancer;

- have disease of the gallbladder;
- have a condition called systemic lupus erythematosus (SLE).

What do I do if I miss a pill?

Most combined pills are taken for 21 days and then you have a break for 7 days when you will have a withdrawal bleed. It is important that you remember to start taking the pill again on time. Some pill packs have dummy (sugar) pills for you to take on your pill-free week so that it is just easier to remember. If you think you may find it difficult to start again after the pill-free week it is worth talking to your doctor about one of these brands.

If you miss a pill, your chances of becoming pregnant will depend on where in the pack you are and how many pills were missed. If you miss just one pill, you should take it as soon as you realize and shouldn't need to take any other action. If you miss two or more pills, take the last one you should have taken as soon as you realize but don't worry about the other missed pills and continue the rest of the pack as normal. You are at risk of becoming pregnant though, so you should use an additional form of contraception for the next seven days and if you have had sex during the time that you missed the pills you will need post-coital emergency contraception. If there are seven or fewer pills left in the pack after your missed pills, continue the pack and run straight into the next one without a pill-free interval.

Remember if you have sickness or diarrhoea this may affect the absorption of your pill and you should continue taking the pill, but consider this in the same way as potentially missing a pill. Some medications and the herbal remedy St John's wort can also affect the way the pill works so always check with your doctor.

The progesterone-only pill (POCP)

The progesterone-only pill is sometimes also referred to as the 'mini pill'. Nothing to do with size, but it contains just one hormone – progesterone. It is taken every day without the pill-free interval and works by thickening mucus and thinning the lining of the womb.

One type (Cerazette) also prevents ovulation. Most mini pills need to be taken within three hours of the same time every day but because of its action on ovulation, Cerazette has the same 12 hour window as the combined pill. It is 99 per cent effective and has fewer serious side effects than the COCP. However, some women find their bleeding becomes less predictable. You should start taking the mini pill in exactly the same was as the COCP and the same rules apply in terms of how quickly you will be protected. Unlike the combined pill, it is fine to use this form of contraception while breastfeeding as it is only the oestrogen component that is transferred in breast milk.

The contraceptive patch

The contraceptive patch has the same hormones as the COCP so many of the same rules apply. It is a thin, beige-coloured patch about 5 cm square that is applied to the skin once a week. It is very effective but research has shown that it may be less so for women weighing more than 90 kilograms (14 stone). Because the hormones are absorbed directly through the skin, the patch is not affected by diarrhoea or vomiting. Some women get skin irritation at the site of the patch but, if you vary where you place it each week, you may be able to minimize this. There appears to be a slightly higher risk of blood clots when using the patch compared to the COCP.

Contraceptive vaginal ring

This is a small see-through ring about 5 cm in diameter. It contains the same hormones as the combined pill so there are similar side effects, but it is placed into the vagina and left in situ for three weeks so doesn't require you to remember to take a pill every morning. At the end of three weeks, you remove the ring and replace it. It is similarly effective to the combined pill and because the hormone is absorbed directly there is no problem with diarrhoea and vomiting. However, some women and or their partners say it can cause irritation during intercourse.

Barrier methods

Male condoms

Male condoms are made of latex (rubber) or a plastic called polyurethane. They fit over the erect penis and are about 98 per cent effective as a contraceptive. It is important to use the correct size of condom. Most men will be fine using a standard size condom as the size of the erect penis doesn't usually vary much, average being 5.5 to 6.5 inches, but there are larger and smaller options available. If a condom is used properly, the man should pull out of the vagina after he has ejaculated, holding the condom in place before the penis becomes flaccid again, so as to ensure no semen enters the vagina. Oil-based products such as body lotions can also weaken latex condoms, which could make them less effective. The great advantage of condoms over the pills and patches is that they also protect against sexually transmitted diseases.

The female condom

The female condom is made of polyurethane and is less popular and less effective at just 95 per cent effective. The one advantage that it has over the male condom is that it can be put in any time before sex and doesn't require the penis to be erect first. It is easy for the female condom to slip if not placed properly.

Diaphragms and caps

Diaphragms and caps fit inside the vagina to cover the cervix and prevent sperm entering the womb. Diaphragms are dome shaped and made of latex or silicone. Caps are made of the same material but are smaller in size. They are 92–6 per cent effective. They are used with a spermicide. If you want to use either of these as a form of contraceptive, you will be taught how to place the device yourself and you will be asked to go away and practise but not to rely on it as a form of contraception until you have been back to your GP or Family Planning Clinic with it in place so that the doctor or nurse can check that you have fitted it correctly. You can put a diaphragm or cap in any time up to three hours before intercourse but it must stay in for at least six hours after intercourse. If your cap or diaphragm has been in place for more than three hours before intercourse, you should use extra spermicide.

Long-acting reversible contraceptives (LARCs)

All the long-acting reversible contraceptives have the advantage that once fitted, you don't need to think about contraception for weeks or even years. They just do their thing.

Contraceptive injections

Contraceptive injections are over 99 per cent effective. They work by thickening cervical mucus and thinning the lining of the womb. They are usually injected into your buttock and need to be repeated every 8 or 13 weeks depending on the type of injection you have. Some women find that their bleeding become unpredictable especially after the first injection but most women will actually stop their periods altogether using the injection. The injection can cause weight gain in some women and, it seems, particularly in women under 18 who are already overweight.

What are the side effects of the injection?

Irregular bleeding is quite common in the early stages and weight gain can sometimes be an issue. We always stress that it is important that women attend on time for repeat injections and there is no long-term risk to fertility but there can be a delay of up to a year when coming off the injection before periods start again and fertility is completely back to normal. It is also possible to get side effects from the hormone, which include acne, hair loss, mood swings, loss of libido and headaches. Long term it is possible that the injection can affect your oestrogen levels and put you at risk of osteoporosis (brittle bones). If you have other risk factors for this disease such as low weight, excess alcohol intake, a positive family history, long-term use of steroids, cigarette smoking or thyroid disease, then your doctor may suggest an alternative form of contraception. We don't recommend routinely scanning to check the health of your bones before starting the injection.

Contraceptive implants

This contraceptive is a matchstick-sized rod that is placed under the skin in your upper arm under local anaesthetic. It slowly releases small amounts of progesterone and works for three years before it needs replacing. It is over 99 per cent effective. It works by stopping ovulation, thickening cervical mucus and thinning the lining of the womb. Your fertility will return to normal as soon as it is removed. It is removed under local anaesthetic. Some women get progestogenic side effects such as acne, hair loss and mood swings but it is generally well tolerated. It is common to have some erratic bleeding initially. This usually settles and your doctor can prescribe hormone pills to regulate things if it is a nuisance.

Intra-uterine devices (coils or IUDs)

IUDs are small plastic or copper devices that are placed through the neck of the womb or the cervix into the uterus. There are several different types available that last for 5 to 10 years depending on the type before they need replacing. If you are over 40 when you have an IUD fitted, it will last through to the menopause. An IUD can be fitted by your GP or Family Planning Clinic and they are over 99 per cent effective. It works as soon as it is put in and your fertility will return as soon as it is removed. It can be fitted anywhere in your cycle but we try to fit an IUD towards the end or just after a period as this is when the cervix is naturally a little opened to allow menstrual blood to flow. Some women find their periods are heavier with an IUD but some of this may also be because a lot of women go from using the COCP (where periods are lighter) to an IUD so we are not always comparing like with like.

Are there any risks with an IUD?

There is a tiny risk of perforating the uterus when the IUD is fitted. Thankfully this is very rare. There is also a small risk of infection in the first three weeks after an IUD is fitted and some women expel the IUD after it has been fitted. If this is going to happen, it usually happens soon after fitting. If you do become pregnant while using the IUD, there is also a slight risk of developing an ectopic pregnancy – a pregnancy that forms in your tubes rather than in the womb. An IUD can be removed very quickly in clinic.

The intra-uterine system (IUS)

This is a small plastic device that is fitted in exactly the same way as the IUD but it secretes tiny amount of progesterone into the womb. The total hormone level is about the same as taking two mini pills a week. There are two types and they are over 99 per cent effective. An IUS works by thickening the cervical mucus and thinning the lining of the womb. In some women it also prevents ovulation. It works for five years and your fertility returns to normal as soon as it is removed. Even though the dose of hormone is very low, some women notice headaches, acne and breast tenderness but, in my experience, the thing that most women mention is erratic bleeding in the early days. This can be a persistent problem for some women but for most it settles over about six months and after that periods often become lighter or stop altogether.

Sterilization

Male sterilization (vasectomy)

Vasectomy involves cutting, clipping or sealing the tubes that carry sperm from the testicles to the penis ready for ejaculation. It is a very effective form of contraception but not 100 per cent as many people assume. About 1 in 2000 vasectomies fail. Vasectomy is available on the NHS but reversal is not, so it is important that you are absolutely certain, no matter how your circumstances may change, that you have completed your family and that involves considering some pretty extreme situations like the death of a partner or child or a windfall of a life-changing amount of money. By law, you don't need your partner's consent to be sterilized but many doctors are reluctant to go ahead unless it is a joint decision.

A vasectomy is done under local anaesthetic and a tiny puncture is made in each side of your scrotum. The tubes are then cut and closed off either by tying them or by using heat to seal them. Often the wound is so small that you don't even need stitches and you will be free to go home the same day. You may feel a bit bruised for a few days and you must continue to use contraception when you are sexually active again until your follow up appointment, which will be about three months later. This is to ensure that any sperm in the tubes have cleared. At that stage you will be asked to provide a sample of ejaculate to check that no sperm are present. You may have to provide more than one sample. As soon as the doctors are happy that there is no longer any sperm in your ejaculate, you no longer need to use any other contraception.

Female sterilization

Female sterilization is a bigger operation as it involves a general anaesthetic. It is usually done by keyhole surgery and the fallopian tubes are cut and tied or sealed in a similar way. This form of sterilization is less effective than male sterilization – 1 in 200 female sterilizations fail and in fact now that we have the IUS, we routinely offer this as an alternative as it is so effective and has the benefit of being easily reversible if circumstances change. There is also now a technique that allows the tubes to be blocked by inserting a tiny titanium coil into the fallopian tubes. This can be done through the cervix so doesn't require any incisions.

Natural methods

Natural family planning requires a woman to be in tune with her body such that she can recognize the signs building up to and around ovulation and avoid intercourse at these times. The fertile period can be as long as 8 or 9 days because sperm can live for seven days and, just occasionally, a second egg may be produced up to 24 hours after the first. These are the signs a woman needs to look for:

- *Body temperature* If you record your body temperature before you get out of bed each day and before you have anything to eat or drink, you will notice that at the time of ovulation your temperature will rise very slightly, about 0.2 degrees centigrade (0.4 degrees Fahrenheit). This is when you are fertile. Your fertile time ends when your temperature has been higher for three days in a row after six days of it being lower.
- *Cervical secretions* become clearer and wetter just before ovulation, a bit like the consistency of raw egg white. This is your fertile time. After ovulation the secretions become thicker and sticky. When they have been like this for three days you are no longer in your fertile phase.
- *Cervical changes* Your cervix will feel slightly higher in the vagina and become softer and slightly open around the time of ovulation, which indicates your fertile time.

As you can see these changes are quite subtle and it usually takes women several months to recognize the signs reliably, but if used properly natural methods can be very effective and there are also now monitors that you can buy that measure urinary hormones to help you predict your fertile times.

Emergency contraception

If you have had unprotected sex or you think your contraception has failed, there are three options available to you to help prevent pregnancy. Two are pills (Levonelle and ellaOne) and the third is an IUD. You can go to any GP, Family Planning Clinic or walk-in centre to access emergency contraception although they may not provide all options. Levonelle is also available over the counter at pharmacies and in some minor injuries units and Accident and Emergency centres.

- Levonelle can be taken any time up to 72 hours after unprotected sex, but the sooner it is taken after the intercourse, the more effective it is.

- ellaOne can be taken any time up to 120 hours after unprotected intercourse.
- An IUD can be fitted any time up to 120 hours after intercourse.

All are effective if taken or used properly, but none of these are absolutely 100 per cent so if your next period is delayed or you develop symptoms suggestive of pregnancy, such as breast swelling and tenderness, fatigue, urinating more frequently, and headaches or nausea, it is important that you do a pregnancy test.

7
Fertility

Eight out of ten couples trying to conceive will do so within the first year as long as they are not using contraception and they are having sex every two to three days. Of those couples who are not pregnant at the end of that year, half will conceive within the next year. In other words, 90 per cent of couples should conceive within two years of trying.

The 10 per cent of couples that have not fallen pregnant may require investigation. In about a quarter of these cases we don't find a specific cause but when we do, the main causes are:

- male problems, such as low sperm count (25 per cent);
- ovulation problems (25 per cent);
- tubal problems, such as blocked fallopian tubes (20 per cent);
- uterine problems (10 per cent).

In around 40 per cent of cases there is a mixture of male and female problems.

What can I do to improve my fertility?

Making sure that you are in good health will improve your fertility and there are a number of lifestyle issues which should be addressed.

- *Weight* Women whose body mass index (BMI) is less than 19 may not be ovulating and gaining weight may help. You can calculate your BMI by dividing your weight (in kilograms) by the square of your height (in metres). Being overweight (BMI greater than 25) can also affect both male and female fertility. Sperm quality and quantity is adversely affected by weight and the greater the amount of excess weight the more significant the impact on sperm. Ovulation is also affected by weight, so ideally both couples should aim for a BMI between 19 and 25.

- *Smoking* impairs female fertility and sperm production.
- *Alcohol* Women trying to conceive should limit their alcohol intake to 1 or 2 units of alcohol once or twice a week and should avoid getting drunk. We are not sure about the effects of moderate alcohol consumption on male fertility but heavy drinking undoubtedly has an effect on testosterone levels and male fertility.
- *Street drugs* Cannabis can impair ovulation and cocaine can have an effect on the tubes, causing infertility. In men anabolic steroids, cannabis, cocaine, heroin and amphetamines can all adversely affect fertility.
- *Prescribed medication* Some prescription medications can affect fertility. Don't ever stop a prescription medicine without speaking to your doctor first, but it is worth checking before you try to conceive to see if your medication may need to be changed.
- *Clothing* If a man is thought to have a problem that might affect his fertility, it is important he wears loosely fitted clothing to keep the testicles cool. Testicles hang outside the body because they need to be cool to ensure good sperm production.

When should I see my doctor?

If you have been having regular unprotected sex for a year without success, it is worth seeing your GP, who may do some initial blood tests and a semen analysis. If you are a woman over 35 or have had known problems in the past, you should go sooner.

Female fertility problems

Problems with ovulation

Absent periods (amenorrhoea)

Amenorrhoea can be primary (periods never start) or secondary (periods were normal but have now stopped). There are lots of reasons why periods stop. Probably the most common is pregnancy and the second the menopause and while the average age for the menopause in the UK is 50–52, it is possible to go through the change much earlier. A menopause before 40 is described as a premature menopause and I have met women in their twenties who are going through 'the change'. Your GP will be able to test for this with blood tests.

It is common to find there is a delay in periods restarting after being on the combined pill. Periods usually resume within 6 months though, and if they don't, other possibilities should be checked out.

Significant weight loss will also stop periods as nature considers very thin women to be unable to carry a healthy pregnancy so shuts down your hormones, which is why anorexic girls and some very thin athletes stop their periods. In these cases, maintaining a healthy body weight and moderating exercise may be all that you need to do to improve your fertility.

Polycystic ovary syndrome (PCOS)

The diagnosis of polycystic ovary syndrome is made in women who have at least two of the following three problems:

- raised testosterone levels; all women have small amounts of the male hormone testosterone but in PCOS these levels are raised;
- multiple cysts (at least 12) in the ovaries;
- anovulatory cycles, i.e. menstrual cycles where ovulation does not occur.

The underlying problems explain the wide variety of symptoms associated with the syndrome. The raised testosterone levels may cause acne, unwanted facial or body hair and thinning of the scalp hair. It is the anovulatory cycles that may lead to erratic periods and problems with fertility.

PCOS sufferers become resistant to insulin, meaning that insulin levels rise, and high insulin levels lead to weight gain. This becomes something of a vicious circle as excess fat makes insulin resistance worse and circulating insulin levels rise further still, potentially meaning further weight gain. In the long term, PCOS increases the risk of developing type 2 diabetes, high blood pressure and high cholesterol. Unsurprisingly, lots of women with PCOS develop issues with low self-esteem and some become depressed.

How is PCOS treated?

It is tough for women with PCOS to lose weight because of the high circulating insulin levels but weight loss is vital as it will improve so many of the associated symptoms. Losing weight helps with fertility issues but some women require a procedure to drill into the ovaries to help with fertility.

Problems of the cervix, uterus or tubes

Infection

Undiagnosed sexually transmitted infections such as chlamydia or gonorrhoea, which have consequently been left untreated, can lead to infection in the fallopian tubes causing them to be damaged. It is one of the reasons we are so keen to detect sexually transmitted infections (see Chapter 8). I have seen too many young women who were completely unaware that they had had chlamydia, for example, only to discover years later that their tubes have been irreversibly damaged leaving them with fertility problems.

Infection can also follow any gynaecological procedure, a miscarriage or after childbirth. Infection can also damage the womb causing adhesions. This is called Asherman's syndrome.

Abnormalities of the uterus

Some women are born with a septum in the uterus or even with what is called a bicornuate uterus. These abnormalities of shape shouldn't generally cause a problem with conception but they may predispose to miscarriage or premature birth.

Abnormalities with the cervix

Problems with the cervix are usually as a result of previous treatment such as a cone biopsy. Some couples do experience fertility problems as a result of what is called cervical mucus hostility to sperm.

Male fertility problems

A low sperm count is defined as less than 15 million sperm per millilitre of semen (see What tests will my doctor do?). A low sperm factor is the sole problem in about one in five couples struggling to conceive and contributes to the problem in a further 25 per cent of couples. We test semen more than once if there is an abnormality as about one in ten samples may come back as abnormal on the first test, but subsequent testing shows a normal result.

What causes a low sperm count?

There are a number of different causes and these include:

- *Hormonal problems* If there is a hormonal imbalance where the testicles produce little or no testosterone, then sperm production is impaired.
- *Chromosomal problems* There is an inherited genetic condition known as Kleinfelter's Syndrome, where instead of having the normal XY chromosomal make up, the man has XXY and this is associated with low testosterone levels and small testes.
- *Anatomical problems* The most common of these is an undescended testicle. The testicles develop in the abdomen in the foetus and move down into the scrotal sac. If they fail to do this and remain in the abdomen they are kept warm and sperm production is impaired. Some boys are also born with abnormalities of the tubes that deliver sperm to the ejaculate.
- *Infections* Chlamydia and gonorrhoea may not produce symptoms but can affect sperm production, which is why it is so important that they are detected and treated (see Chapter 8).

Infection of the prostate gland, known as prostatitis, has a similar effect.

- *Trauma* This may be through injury or surgery. Both can affect sperm production.
- *Medication* Some prescription medication, such as chemotherapy, some antibiotics and ulcer medications, can affect sperm production as well as many street drugs including anabolic steroids and other substances of misuse.
- *Chemicals* Exposure to some pesticides is thought to adversely effect sperm production.
- *Varicocele* This is a collection of dilated veins in the testicle. The increased blood supply through these veins results in a rise in temperature, which can affect spermatogenesis.

What tests will my doctor do?

If there is a problem with conceiving it is always better to be seen as a couple so that the doctor can explain things to both of you at every step of the way. Initial tests will include a Day 21 blood test for the woman and a semen analysis for the man.

- *Day 21 test* The Day 21 progesterone test assumes a regular 28 day cycle. The blood test should be done 7 days before the onset of a period, so if your cycle is 21 days it would be taken on day 14 (counting the first day of bleeding as day 1) and if you have a 35 day cycle it would be taken on day 28. The thinking is that you should ovulate 14 days before a period and after ovulation your progesterone levels should rise. So if we take a blood test 7 days after assumed ovulation we are looking for a progesterone level over 30. If it is less than 30, it suggests you probably haven't ovulated in that cycle or that we got the timing wrong so it would be repeated on subsequent cycles. If periods are very irregular your GP will also test for other hormones called follicle stimulating hormone (FSH) and luteinizing hormone (LH), which may give an indication of ovarian failure or polycystic ovarian syndrome (PCOS).

- *Semen analysis* A semen sample has to be collected by masturbation and not into a condom as many condoms contain spermicide, which will of course affect the result, and it should be produced after three days of sexual abstinence. It has to be delivered to the laboratory ideally within an hour of production. In most instances this will mean that you will have to liaise with the laboratory to prearrange a delivery time.

A normal result would show these approximate results:

- volume, 1.5 millilitres;
- total sperm number, 39 million sperm;
- 40 per cent motile sperm;
- 58 per cent live sperm;
- 4 per cent normal sperm forms.

If these tests show a specific problem then you will be referred for further investigation or treatment. Other tests may include:

- Testicular biopsy, a test in which a small sample of tissue is removed from the testicle under local anaesthetic. The tissue is analyzed under a microscope to assess sperm production.
- Hysterosalpingogram, where dye is injected through the cervix into the uterine cavity and can be viewed radiologically to check that it can flow through the fallopian tubes, suggesting that they are not blocked.
- Laparoscopy and dye test, where the dye is injected through the cervix and can be viewed through keyhole surgery. This test also allows the specialist to check for endometrial deposits as seen in endometriosis (see Chapter 9).
- Ovarian reserve testing, which is basically an assessment of how many eggs a woman has left. Using a combination of ultrasound and blood tests, specialists can predict the likelihood of response to in vitro fertilization (IVF) if couples are considering this option.

8

Sexually transmitted infections (STIs)

Vaginal discharge

All women will experience vaginal discharge. Not only are we all different but vaginal discharge varies throughout the cycle in each woman and what is normal for one woman may not be acceptable for another. It is thought that around one in ten women will consult their GP during their lifetime with concerns over vaginal discharge. Sometimes this will simply be looking for reassurance that everything is healthy but sometimes it may be related to a problem that needs further investigation or treatment.

What is normal vaginal discharge?

Normal vaginal discharge is colourless or white, although it may become more yellow on exposure to air as a result of oxidation. It should not be blood stained and should not have an odour. It tends to become thicker and more profuse following ovulation and some women using oral contraception or the coil may notice an increase in the amount of discharge they produce. A change in your vaginal secretions doesn't necessarily mean infection. A cervical erosion or polyp can cause increased discharge and a foreign body in the vagina – most commonly a forgotten tampon – is a relatively common cause of discharge. It can also be a sign of a cancer but this is extremely rare and infective causes are much more likely.

Thrush

Thrush is caused by a yeast called *Candida albicans* which is actually present in the vagina of 20 per cent of women without causing symptoms. If it does cause symptoms it is likely to cause soreness and itching in the vagina and vulva and a cottage cheese-like discharge, or a red sore rash on the penis, usually around the glans, in men.

Who gets thrush?

Thrush is extremely common and there may be no obvious reason why some women suffer but it is more common in:

- *Diabetes* Diabetics with poor diabetic control will have high blood sugar levels that provide the perfect environment for thrush to thrive. In fact, if a woman presents with recurrent thrush she should always be tested for undiagnosed diabetes.
- *Pregnancy* Hormonal changes in pregnancy can increase the likelihood of developing thrush.
- *Antibiotics* It is normal to have bacteria in our vaginas and, when in the right balance, these bacteria play a role in keeping the vagina clean and healthy. If you have antibiotics for an infection elsewhere in the body, that can reduce the amount of bacteria in your vagina meaning that the yeast that causes thrush can proliferate to cause symptoms.
- *Steroids* Taking steroids increases the likelihood of developing thrush.
- *Immune problems* AIDS or taking drugs to damp down your immune system, for other conditions you may have, can make you more prone to thrush.

Contrary to popular belief, taking the combined oral contraceptive pill has not been proven to make you more prone to thrush but if I see a woman plagued with recurrent thrush who is using the combined pill, I sometimes suggest an alternative form of contraception and occasionally it does the trick.

Will I have to have a swab test?

I don't always swab people with symptoms of thrush. If you have had it before and recognize the symptoms and are in a monogamous relationship, you may simply need the treatment, which can come in the form of creams, vaginal pessaries for women or tablets.

If, however, there is any possibility of a sexually transmitted infection your doctor will want to check this out with a swab test.

What can I do to prevent thrush developing?

If you suffer with recurrent thrush, make sure you only use underwear made with natural fibres. Avoid man-made fibres, which are likely to make you sweat, and, wherever possible, keep clothing loose. Try to avoid any perfumed products as this will alter the naturally acidic environment of the vagina and mean that the yeast can thrive. The yeast that causes thrush grows in the bowel so after going to the toilet always wipe front to back to avoid encouraging the yeast forward to the vaginal opening. Thrush is not a sexually transmitted infection but some women notice flares after sexual intercourse – if this is you, make sure you use plenty of lubricant during sex to reduce any trauma to the delicate vaginal skin. I often recommend a daily probiotic to maintain good gut health and keep the yeast in balance too. If you suffer with recurrent thrush your doctor may suggest a longer course of treatment in the form of an anti-fungal tablet taken once a week for four weeks.

Bacterial vaginosis

Just as thrush is caused by an overgrowth of yeast, bacterial vaginosis (BV) is caused by an overgrowth of a bacteria called *Gardnerella vaginalis* that occurs naturally in the vagina. It is actually twice as common as thrush although in my experience many women have never heard of it and it is important to know of its existence. I have met so many women over the years who have been self-treating what they presume to be thrush when in fact it is BV.

How can I tell the difference between thrush and BV?

The only way to be absolutely sure is to have a swab test, but there are some characteristic differences. The discharge of thrush tends to be thick and white, like cottage cheese, while the discharge of BV is likely to be more watery and grey; however, the main difference is the odour. The discharge of BV has a fishy odour which women find extremely embarrassing and distressing. Itching is much more a symptom of thrush than BV.

How is BV treated?

Unlike thrush, BV is treated with antibiotics either by mouth or as a vaginal cream. This can, of course, mean you are more prone to thrush and I have met some poor women who seem to oscillate between the two infections. In these women, I recommend using a lactic acid gel inserted into the vagina to maintain a healthy vaginal pH and keep the bacteria in balance. It is particularly important to treat BV in pregnant women as it has been linked to miscarriage and premature birth.

Chlamydia

Chlamydia can cause vaginal or penile discharge, but perhaps the first thing to say is that at least 70 per cent of women and 50 per cent of men with chlamydia will have no symptoms at all and those that do may only have a mild discharge and/or pain or burning when passing urine. Other symptoms include bleeding between periods and pelvic or lower abdominal pain. In fact if a woman presents to me with bleeding between periods, which cannot be explained by missed pills or any other obvious cause, it is chlamydia until proved otherwise.

Unfortunately chlamydia is so prevalent because it often goes unrecognized and I have met too many women over the years who only discover they have been infected when they are trying for a baby and discover that previously undiagnosed chlamydia has resulted in blocked fallopian tubes leading to infertility. Like all things, prevention is better than cure – practising safe sex by using a barrier method of contraception with new sexual partners will protect you from this disease. If you have had unprotected sex and think you could be at risk, you should see your GP or any sexual health clinic for a swab and/or urine test. If chlamydia is confirmed, you will be given a short course of antibiotics. Your partner and all other sexual partners in the last six months should also be tested.

Gonorrhoea

While gonorrhoea can, like chlamydia, go undetected, it is more likely to cause symptoms. Around 50 per cent of women with gonorrhoea will notice a change in their vaginal discharge and about one in four may notice pain in the lower abdomen. Just like chlamydia, if gonorrhoea is left untreated it can have implications for future fertility, so if you know you have been at possible risk it is worth getting it checked out. Symptoms in men are much more common. About nine out of ten infected men will notice a fluid discharge from the penis which usually develops 5 to 7 days after infection. There may also be some redness around the urethral opening at the end of the penis. Complications are less common in men but occasionally a narrowing of the urethra (the tube that allows urine to flow from the bladder out through the penis) can occur. This is called a urethral stricture. Gonorrhoea can be diagnosed with a simple swab or urine test and is easily treated with antibiotics.

Trichomoniasis

The discharge of trichomoniasis is frothy and may be green or yellow in colour. It may smell fishy just like bacterial vaginosis but, unlike BV, soreness and irritation can be quite intense. Just like chlamydia and gonorrhoea, it may show no symptoms at all, especially in men. It is easily treated with antibiotics and it is important that it is treated because the presence of trichomoniasis can increase your risk of contracting HIV and if caught during pregnancy it increases the risk of premature labour.

Genital warts

Genital warts remain the most common sexually transmitted infection. They are caused by infection with human papilloma virus (HPV) types 6 and 11. These are not the strains of HPV that are implicated in cervical and other forms of cancer but they are covered by the vaccine that is currently offered to all 12 and 13 year old girls so we will hopefully see a fall in the incidence of warts in the future. Genital warts are spread by skin to skin contact, so the use of condoms doesn't offer full protection. The warts can develop a few weeks after contact but can also be noticed for the first time several years after infection, so a recent onset of warts doesn't necessarily mean a partner has been unfaithful!

Small warts may be treated by the application of creams or ointments for a few days each week; sometimes for several weeks. They can be frozen off by cryotherapy, or removed by heat using electrocautery. They can also be removed surgically under local anaesthetic or by using a laser.

Genital herpes

Genital herpes is the most common cause of ulcers on the genitals and these can be extremely painful. There are two types of herpes simplex virus – types 1 and 2. Usually, type 1 causes cold sores and type 2 causes genital ulceration, but there is quite a bit of overlap and either type can cause either symptom.

The first episode of herpes often involves multiple ulcers, which are painful and can last up to three weeks. These can be treated with antiviral medication on prescription. Subsequent attacks are thankfully typically less severe and often heralded by a tingling sensation. If antiviral cream available over the counter is used at this stage, the blisters can be avoided. Once an individual has contracted herpes, the infection never completely clears from the body. The virus crawls back up the nerve endings and lays dormant. In some people, there will never be a recurrence but for others, recurrences are a regular problem. They tend to flare when you are run down or stressed and after exposure to ultra violet light. During a flare up, you will be highly infectious and should avoid sexual intercourse. Once the lesions have healed you are of very low infectivity, although it is still possible to pass the virus on so condoms should be used all the time.

Syphilis

Syphilis is a sexually transmitted infection caused by a bacteria called *Treponema pallidum*. The first stage of the disease, known as primary syphilis, causes painless ulcers on the genital area. These usually occur two to three weeks after the infection was caught and are highly infectious. They can take up to six weeks to heal. The second stage, known as secondary syphilis, causes a painless non-itchy pink or red rash all over the body. There may also be warty-like lesions around the genitals which can easily be mistaken for warts and white patches on the roof of the mouth along with patchy hair loss. The third stage, or tertiary syphilis, is very rare in the UK and occurs several years later causing damage to the heart, bones, brain and nervous system. Syphilis is easily treated with antibiotic injections. In primary and secondary syphilis this treatment will completely cure the condition. You can also cure tertiary syphilis quickly, but you cannot reverse the damage already done to the heart, bones, brain and nerves.

Pubic lice (*Phthirus pubis*)

Sometimes also called crabs, pubic lice are tiny grey or brown insects smaller than the head of a match. They can live in any hairy area but they like thick hair so tend to congregate in pubic hair. They are spread by direct contact so it is possible to contract lice through intimate physical contact without actually having intercourse. They cause intense itching, although this may not develop for a couple of weeks after infection and the itch is usually worse at night when the lice feed on blood in the skin. They are treated with creams and lotions and treatment should be repeated a week later to ensure any eggs which could have hatched are also killed. You should also wash all bed linen and underwear on a hot wash. Always ask any sexual partners to check themselves closely for lice and don't be concerned if the itching persists for a few days after treatment as it can take a little while to settle.

Scabies (*Sarcoptes scabiei*)

Scabies is caused by a tiny mite, which is only just visible to the naked eye. The female mites tunnel under the skin to lay their eggs. The eggs hatch after three or four days and grow into adult mites over the next ten to 15 days. The main symptom is that of extreme itching, which is actually caused not so much by the presence of the mite but by our own immune reaction to the saliva and faeces produced by the mites. Scabies can be passed from person to person by skin to skin contact and, along with intense itching, it may be possible to see the burrows themselves, which look like fine silvery or brown lines up to a centimetre long. Patients also often develop a widespread red blotchy rash.

Scabies is common, affecting about one in a thousand people every month, but thankfully it is easily treated with creams and lotions from the chemist. It is important to follow the instructions and to treat all household members. All clothing, towels and bed linen should be washed on a hot wash and treatment should be repeated a week later.

HIV & AIDS

HIV stands for human immunodeficiency virus. It is a virus that lives in the white cells in our blood. The white cells are the cells that fight infection but they can't kill the HIV virus because it keeps changing before the white cells have had a chance to fight it. There are over 100,000 people in the UK living with HIV and most of them are men who have sex with men.

AIDS stands for acquired immunodeficiency syndrome. It is a collection of illnesses that some (not all) people infected with HIV can get. The terms HIV & AIDS are sometimes used interchangeably but that is not strictly correct.

How do you contract HIV?

The HIV virus is passed on in bodily fluids, namely blood, semen and vaginal secretions. It is possible to pass the virus on even if the person has no symptoms and has not developed AIDS. Vaginal or anal sex is the commonest way to contract HIV and in fact accounts for about 95 per cent of cases. Oral sex also carries a risk but much less so unless there is a break in the mucous membrane lining the mouth in the form of an ulcer or damaged gums. HIV can also be spread by sharing needles or via a needle stick injury.

It is also possible for an HIV positive mother to pass the infection to her unborn child but with appropriate treatment this transmission occurs in fewer than one in a hundred pregnancies.

What are the symptoms of HIV & AIDS?

About 80 per cent of people infected with HIV will notice a fever, sore throat and red rash at the time of infection. They may also feel sick and have diarrhoea or feel tired and headachy and this can last up to three weeks, but to be fair these are common symptoms and could easily be attributed to any number of viral illnesses. After this you may remain symptom free for many years, but during this time the virus may continue to multiply and eventually, if untreated, you will start to develop infections such as shingles, repeated yeast infections or a reoccurrence of an old TB infection. This happens because the immune system is beginning to fail.

It is only in the advanced stages of untreated HIV infection that people start to develop the unusual infections that we associate with AIDS such as pneumocystis pneumonia and unusual fungal and viral infections. It is at this stage that you may also lose lots of weight and develop AIDS dementia and cancers such as Kaposi's sarcoma.

How is HIV & AIDS diagnosed?

Many sexual health clinics will now offer on-the-spot HIV blood tests, meaning that results are available within the hour, but even without this service most people will have a result within a week. In the past a negative test was likely to go against you in the world of insurance but this is no longer the case and it is recommended that gay and bisexual men should be tested every year.

How is HIV treated?

In the 80s, HIV infection was effectively a death sentence but the development of a number of medicines, called anti-retroviral medicines, means the majority of people infected with HIV can continue to live full and active lives. Most people take a combination of anti-retroviral medications to combat the virus at different stages in its replication. Today there is a once daily pill that contains three different medicines.

How can HIV infection be prevented?

Just like anything else, prevention is better than cure, so practising safe sex by always using a condom and not sharing needles is vital in protecting yourself from HIV infection.

Hepatitis B

Hepatitis B is one of many viruses that can cause inflammation in the liver but I include it here because hepatitis B, just like HIV, is spread through bodily fluids such as blood, semen and vaginal secretions. About one in three people in the UK has persistent (chronic) hepatitis B infection. The acute phase of hepatitis B infection may simply manifest as a flu-like illness but in about half of all cases it presents with sickness, vomiting, fatigue and fever. Some, but not all, people also become jaundiced. For 90 per cent of people the virus then clears and there are no more sequelae, but in 10 per cent a chronic form of the infection ensues. Of these, two-thirds of people will remain well and some will clear the virus over the following years. Sadly, the other small minority go on to develop a persistent inflammation and of those some will be at risk of developing cirrhosis of the liver, which is irreversible.

How can hepatitis B infection be prevented?

Practising safe sex and not sharing needles is important in protecting yourself against hepatitis B infection but, unlike HIV, there is also a vaccination available for those at risk.

9

Sexual problems in women

Low libido

This is probably the most common sexual problem that I see in surgery. There are two main different types, which in medicine we refer to as primary low sexual desire and secondary low sexual desire. As the name implies, primary low sexual desire refers to the woman who has never had an interest in sexual activity. There are usually deep-rooted issues behind this – often a woman with primary low sexual desire will have been brought up being told that sex is wrong or dirty and unravelling that can take a lot of time in therapy. Secondary low sexual desire is the more common problem and refers to the woman who has had a healthy sex drive in the past but has lost all interest in recent weeks, months or years. By the time I see women like this in my consulting room it has usually been an issue for months or years and more often than not she has been encouraged to seek help by her partner. The first question to ask yourself is whether you ever have any sexual desire. If you masturbate or have sexual fantasies but have no sexual interest in your partner then you are looking at a relationship issue and that needs to be addressed.

It is common for women to notice a drop in their libido following childbirth and this is down to several factors. Hormones are all over the place. Your body will have changed shape and you may feel less attractive. I always encourage women who are bothered by this to talk to their partners outside of the bedroom. If you are feeling frumpy and your underwear doesn't fit properly then investing in some new underwear that fits and makes you feel more feminine may help you to feel better about yourself. It takes time to regain a pre-pregnancy figure and most of us never return completely to the pre-pregnancy state but remember it is a small price to pay for the wonder that is motherhood and in time you will learn to be comfortable in your new body. You are also likely to be tired. Bed becomes for sleeping in when you are experiencing sleepless nights so don't be too hard on yourself. When your baby starts to sleep through and you actually manage to get some sleep again your libido will return but it is not uncommon for women to notice a fall in their libido for up to a year after childbirth.

Another time in life when I see a lot of women experiencing a fall in their sexual desire is around the time of the menopause. For some women this is an emotional time and comes with a realization that they are getting older, which influences how they feel sexually. Vaginal dryness is also extremely common around this time and can make sex uncomfortable or sometimes even painful. Let's face it – sex is supposed to be fun and if it hurts then it is completely natural to go off the idea! The sadness for me is that so few women report this symptom. More often than not it is a conversation that we have when I notice the tissues of the vagina look a little thin and dry and I ask the question directly. I am usually given one of several responses – 'I can't remember the last time we had sex', 'Yes, it is actually but my husband is very understanding' or 'Yes, it's a bit of an issue actually' and yet very few women proactively come in to ask for help because they assume it is just something they have to put up with as they get older. NO!

Oestrogen pessaries or vaginal cream are very effective at treating this and don't carry the risks of conventional hormone replacement therapy (HRT) as they only work locally in the vagina. When they are first used some hormone does get absorbed into the body through the thin vaginal tissues but as they start to work, the vaginal tissues plump up and become lubricated again and this prevents the absorption of hormone into the body. So it is not uncommon to notice some hormonal symptoms such as breast tenderness and bloating in the early stages but this will subside as the pessaries or cream start to work. Some women really don't want to consider anything hormonal but there are plenty of slow-release lubricants available to help alleviate the problem and your pharmacist will be able to advise. Pharmacies have confidential consulting rooms now so all you have to do is to ask to speak the pharmacist privately. You don't have to talk about this over the counter in front of other people.

Pain during intercourse

Pain during intercourse is a common problem and to identify the cause, your doctor will want to know three things.

- Is the pain at the entrance to the vagina?
- Is the pain felt deep inside?
- Is intercourse painful all the time or just in certain positions?

Pain at the entrance to the vagina can be due to a condition called vaginismus (see page 65) where the muscles around the entrance go into spasm as soon as penetration is attempted. It can also be due to a condition called vulvodynia where the tissues around the entrance become over sensitive, often triggered by an infection, which may be something as simple as thrush. This can be treated with creams available on prescription from your GP. Sometimes there is a small tear to explain the pain, or scar tissue that is not as elastic as healthy vaginal tissue. This can happen following a tear or an episiotomy during childbirth. If there is scar tissue, your doctor may suggest you see a gynaecologist to discuss the option of excising the scar and refashioning it, which often gives good results.

Pain deeper in the vagina which is only felt in certain positions is likely to be due to very deep penetration and can be managed by explaining this to your partner and avoiding those positions. If it occurs during all sexual activity it is more likely to be related to a problem in the pelvis such as endometriosis or chronic pelvic inflammatory disease. It surprises women to know that sometimes it can be due to irritable bowel syndrome (see page 63). The important thing is that you shouldn't put up with it. Once your doctor has worked out what is causing the pain he or she will be able to help you so make that appointment.

Chronic pelvic pain is a miserable condition and I have seen it wreck lives and relationships. Because there are a number of different causes, sadly it can take a long while to reach a diagnosis. If this is happening to you it is worth spending some time thinking about your symptoms before you visit your doctor so that you can give as clear a story as possible of how it affects you.

Ask yourself the simple questions below and jot down your answers.

- Where do you feel the pain?
- Does it spread anywhere else?
- What makes it worse or better?
- Is it linked to your periods and if so how?
- Is it linked to intercourse?
- Do you have any associated vaginal discharge?
- Are there any urinary symptoms?
- Are there any bowel symptoms?

What causes chronic pelvic pain?

Pelvic pain can be due to a number of different conditions and your description of your pain will help your doctor to narrow down the possible causes in you, which is why it is important to spend some time thinking about the nature of your pain.

Endometriosis

Pelvic pain caused by endometriosis characteristically starts a couple of days before a period starts and lasts throughout the period. It is felt in the lower abdomen and can go through to the back or radiate down to the thighs. Endometriosis can also be associated with pain on intercourse, especially during deep penetration, and can last for as long as 24 hours after intercourse. We are not sure why this happens but one theory is that penetration causes pressure on endometrial deposits in the pelvis. The pain of endometriosis is related to the menstrual cycle, usually building during the cycle to be at its worst just before and during a period.

If you have a first degree relative (mother, sister or daughter) with the condition you are much more likely – possibly as much as nine times more likely – to have endometriosis. It saddens me to hear that women with endometriosis wait on average for 8 years before finally being given a diagnosis. By spending some time really thinking about your pain, you will hopefully be diagnosed much sooner. I remember being taught that middle class Caucasian women were more likely to have endometriosis. This isn't so but sadly is more likely to be a reflection of the fact that those women are perhaps more likely to persist in their search for an explanation and get the referral to a gynaecologist that they need. Endometriosis cannot be diagnosed with a scan or a blood test. It is made following a procedure called a laparoscopy (a look inside with a telescope) and needs to be done under anaesthetic by a gynaecologist.

Irritable bowel syndrome (IBS)

It may seem odd that I am suddenly talking bowels when we are discussing pelvic pain but in fact IBS is a very common cause of such pain. Food gets from your mouth, through your gut to your rectum by being pushed along by muscular contractions in the gut wall. There is a lot of debate as to whether people with IBS have stronger than normal contractions causing the classic symptoms of cramping abdominal pain, trapped wind and bloating and constipation or diarrhoea, or whether they simply have a heightened sensitivity to normal contractions. I suspect that both factors play a role.

The pain of IBS will differ from other causes of pelvic pain, the most significant factor being the association with bowel movements. So IBS pain may cause associated diarrhoea or constipation and it is often relieved partially or completely after having your bowels open. There may be mucus in the stool and a feeling of not having completely emptied your bowels after going to the toilet. This is called tenesmus. There may be a link to the menstrual cycle, which is why it can be confused with a gynaecological problem.

The hormonal changes just before a period can affect the muscular contractions in the bowel wall. And stress definitely plays a role – the symptoms invariably increase in times of stress and I have many patients who have medication at hand to take when the pressure is on but who manage with simple lifestyle measures such as increasing fluid and altering fibre intake when life is less stressful.

Chronic pelvic inflammatory disease (PID)

Pelvic inflammatory disease is an infection of the womb and fallopian tubes. The most common cause is a sexually transmitted infection such as chlamydia or gonorrhoea but it can also be caused by overgrowth of the normal bacteria living in the vagina. This is more likely after having a baby or after a procedure such as fitting a coil or having a gynaecological operation. The pain of chronic PID can be experienced on one or both sides of the pelvis and is often linked to intercourse because of sensitivity around the cervix. Some patients will give a clear story of having had a sexually transmitted infection but as infections like chlamydia and gonorrhoea are often asymptomatic in the acute phase, it is perfectly possible to have a chronic inflammation without ever having been aware of the initial infection. There may also be an associated vaginal discharge or abnormal vaginal bleeding, which can be anything from heavier than normal periods, to bleeding after sex or bleeding between periods.

PID can be difficult to diagnose as swabs don't always show any bacteria and scans looking for inflamed fallopian tubes may also appear normal, so it is not uncommon to need a laparoscopy to confirm the diagnosis. Treatment is usually with a combination of antibiotics but around one in five women will have a second episode of PID. This is generally because the partner wasn't treated or the course of antibiotics was not completed, so it is important that you follow the instructions of your treatment and that you practise safe sex with any new partners to reduce your risk of further problems.

Trapped ovary syndrome

This is a rare condition occurring in about 1 in 100 women who have had their womb removed (a hysterectomy) but where the ovaries are left in place. It occurs because the ovary gets stuck to the wall of the vagina, causing pain in the pelvis particularly during intercourse. A similar syndrome can occur in women who have had the ovaries removed at the time of hysterectomy. This is called ovarian remnant syndrome and is thought to be due to the presence of some functioning ovarian tissue despite having apparently having had the ovaries removed. Both conditions can be difficult to treat but involve removing the remaining tissue surgically.

Vaginismus

Vaginismus is spasm of the muscles around the entrance to the vagina, which causes pain on attempted penetration. When severe, it makes penetration impossible. Most cases are primary – that is, it has always been a problem – but it can also be secondary; for example, following trauma during intercourse or a bad sexual experience, such as rape. Treatment involves a combination of psychosexual counselling and the use of vaginal dilators. These come in a variety of sizes so that a woman can start by inserting the smallest cone into her vagina by herself in private, and, over time, gradually working up to the larger cones, which are the size of the average erect penis.

Other physical problems which could cause discomfort during intercourse include the following.

Vulval cancer

Cancer can occur anywhere in the body. When it occurs on the vulva it tends to occur on the inner surface of the inner and outer lips known as the labia minora and labia majora, but it can also occur on the skin around the lips of the vulva or in the clitoris. Vulval cancer is thankfully rare – there are around 1,000 new cases each year in the UK – and it almost always develops after the menopause. There is no one specific cause but we do know that there are some things that increase your risk of developing the disease.

What are the risk factors for developing vulval cancer?

- *Age* Vulval cancer is extremely rare in pre-menopausal women. Most cases occur after the age of 55.
- *Human papilloma virus* I have already discussed the role of HPV in the development of cervical cancer and it would seem it plays a similar role in the development of vulval cancer. HPV types 16, 18 and 31 seem to increase the risk of developing a condition called vulval intra-epithelial neoplasia (VIN) and around a third of all vulval cancers develop from VIN. HPV only seems to play a part in developing vulval cancer in approximately 50 per cent of all cases, whereas it is responsible for 99 per cent of cervical cancers.
- *Smoking* depresses the immune system and therefore makes it less likely that you will effectively clear HPV from your system.
- *Lichen sclerosis and lichen planus (pages 67–8)* Both of these conditions cause inflammation and irritation of the skin around the vulva and can lead to vulval cancer in a very small number of women.
- *Genital herpes* Herpes infection is very common and in most cases has no link to cancer. In a very small minority of women it can increase the risk of developing vulval cancer.

What should I look out for?

The most common symptom of vulval cancer is a persistent itch or soreness. Some women describe a burning sensation, especially when passing urine. It may not be a part of your body that you are used to examining but using a mirror either sitting on the floor or with one foot on a chair you can look at the skin around the vulva. Thickened or raised areas, persistent ulcers or areas of discolouration – either darker looking skin or patches of lighter looking skin – should always be checked out. Any unusual swelling or a mole in that area that is changing should also be reported. Most vulval cancers develop in the skin cells themselves but about 4 per cent develop in the pigment cells and may present as a changing mole. The changes you are looking for are any difference in the size, shape or colour or a mole that starts to itch or bleed.

How is vulval cancer treated?

The diagnosis will first be confirmed by taking a small biopsy of tissue under local anaesthetic for examination under a microscope. If you have vulval cancer your specialist will probably then want to arrange various blood tests and scans to assess how far the cancer has spread before deciding on the best treatment for you. You will almost certainly be offered surgery in the first instance unless the cancer is widely spread and your general health is such that surgery may not be the best option for you. Exactly what operation you will have will depend on the size and position of the cancer. Smaller cancers may be treated by removing just the abnormal area and a small amount of surrounding tissue, whereas larger cancers may involve removing the entire vulval area – the labia minora, majora and clitoris. Radiotherapy may be another option – as most vulval cancers develop in skin cells and are squamous cell cancers they are usually sensitive to radiotherapy. Chemotherapy may also be an option.

Lichen sclerosis

Lichen sclerosis affects about 1 in 1000 women, causing itching around the genital area. We don't know what causes it and sadly we don't have a cure as yet. It can last for years, causing a lot of angst and discomfort. It usually starts as small white spots around the vulva that are intensely itchy. Over time these spots may join together to form larger patches of white skin. Because they are so itchy, the trauma from scratching means that the skin may split and bleed and if left untreated the resulting scar tissue may mean that the entrance to the vagina becomes narrower, making intercourse more difficult. Regular use of steroid ointment on prescription from your doctor will alleviate the symptoms but it should be used sparingly – as a rough guide a 30 g tube of steroid ointment should last around three months.

What else can I do to help myself?

If you have lichen sclerosis, try not to scratch the area. So much easier to say than to do, but the more you scratch, the more you traumatize the skin and the worse the itching becomes so you end up in a vicious scratch–itch cycle. Keep your nails short and wear cotton gloves in bed so that you don't damage the skin in your sleep by scratching before you are fully awake. An anti-histamine at night may also help. Avoid anything perfumed in that area – so no bubble baths or perfumed soap as these may irritate the skin further. Use aqueous cream as a soap substitute. It won't lather in the same way but is very effective and helps soothe the skin. Use an emollient such as petroleum jelly on the area before passing urine to protect from the stinging, only wear natural fibres, and wear stockings rather than tights to keep you cool, as sweating increases the itching. If you are aware that sex is becoming uncomfortable you will need to use plenty of lubricant and speak to your doctor about vaginal dilators to keep the area open.

Lichen planus

Lichen planus also causes itching, but it can affect other areas of the body, including the limbs, mouth, nails and scalp, as well as the genitals. Unlike lichen sclerosis it tends to clear up after several months and rarely lasts more than 18 months. Steroid creams will help with symptoms, as will all the self-help measures used to manage lichen sclerosis.

Bartholin's cyst

The Bartholin's glands are small pea-sized glands that sit just inside the vagina and their function is to secrete lubricant fluid during intercourse. Sometimes the ducts that deliver the fluid can become blocked and the cyst develops. Small cysts may not cause any problems at all and although any new lump should be checked out by your doctor, you may not need any specific treatment. Sometimes if the cysts become very large they can be painful and interfere with sex, in which case they may need to be removed surgically (although in about one in five cases, they do recur). If they become sore and inflamed this could suggest infection, which will need antibiotics.

10

Sexual problems in men

Erectile dysfunction (ED)

Erectile dysfunction (or impotence) means the inability to get or maintain an erection sufficient for penetration. It will happen to virtually all men at some point – if they are stressed, overtired or have drunk too much alcohol – but for some men it is a persistent problem and while that can be psychological, in eight out of ten cases there is a physical cause so it is important that it is checked out. It is a very common problem – it is estimated that around half of all men aged between 40 and 70 have a degree of ED and almost three-quarters of men over 70 will suffer.

What causes ED?

In a minority of cases there is purely psychological cause to ED, which may be stress, anxiety, depression or relationship problems. And of course as soon as ED starts to become a problem, even purely from a physical cause, then emotional factors play a part too. These are the some of the physical causes of ED:

- *Circulatory* Reduced blood flow to the penis caused by narrowing of the blood vessels supplying it is by far the most common cause of ED. In fact ED is often the first indicator of other vascular disease.
- *Neurological* Diseases affecting the nervous system like multiple sclerosis or Parkinson's disease can also affect the nerves supplying the penis, resulting in ED. Pressure on the nerves, for example during long distance cycling, can also cause ED, and trauma to the pelvis can likewise be to blame.
- *Hormonal* A lack of testosterone is a rare cause of ED.
- *Medical* Some prescribed medicines and street drugs can cause

ED. If you have recently started a new drug and developed ED it is certainly worth discussing with your GP but don't ever be tempted to stop a prescription drug without talking to your doctor first.

Reduced blood flow to the penis from narrowed arteries accounts for about seven out of ten cases of ED so it worth thinking about that in a little more detail here. The risk factors for this are the same as any other vessel disease.

- *Smoking* The more you smoke, the greater the risk.
- *Obesity* A high fat diet will increase your risk. The risk is highest when the excess weight is carried around the middle. If you took two identical men, same height and same weight, but one man carries his weight around his middle (apple shaped) and the other carries his weight around his hips and thighs (pear shaped), the apple-shaped man would have a greater risk of developing vascular disease than the pear-shaped.
- *Lack of exercise* You should aim to exercise for at least 30 minutes at least five times a week.
- *Hypertension* High blood pressure increases the risk of ED.
- *Cholesterol* Only 20 per cent of our cholesterol is derived from our diets, so even if you eat healthily you could still have a high cholesterol as the other 80 per cent is made up by our bodies.
- *Type 2 diabetes* Not only does type 2 diabetes increase your risk but it actually magnifies the effect of the other risk factors.
- *Alcohol* Consistently drinking more than the recommended 14 units per week for men increases your risk of vascular disease and binge drinking is thought to be the most risky.

The link between ED and other vascular disease is so strong that it is thought that men with ED are twice as likely to have a heart attack and a one in ten increased risk of a stroke so it is certainly worth taking these risk factors seriously.

What will my doctor do?

Your doctor will certainly want to check some blood tests to look at your cholesterol levels and check you out for diabetes as well as liver and kidney function. He or she will check your blood pressure and arrange a tracing of your heart to check that it isn't showing signs of strain.

What treatment can I have?

Your doctor will definitely want to address any risk factors so you may be offered treatment for high blood pressure or high cholesterol if necessary. There are several oral medications available to treat ED, which work by increasing blood flow to the penis. They need to be taken before sexual intercourse and will only work if you are then sexually aroused. You won't get a spontaneous erection without arousal. The tablets are sildenafil (Viagra), tadalafil (Cialis) and vardenafil (Levitra). All these drugs can interact with other prescription medicines so it is important your doctor knows what you are taking before prescribing them.

There are also injections available which are injected into the base of the penis and cause a spontaneous erection, irrespective of whether you have been aroused, within about 15 minutes. These are less popular (for obvious reasons!) since the development of tablets. You can also use a pump, into which you place the flaccid penis and then suck out the air. As this happens it also sucks blood into the penis causing an erection. A rubber band is then placed around the base of the penis to maintain the erection.

Finally some men have a prosthesis implanted in the penis with a valve placed into the scrotum. When pressed this valve allows fluid from a chamber inserted in the abdominal cavity to flow into the prosthesis causing an erection. Pressing another valve allows the fluid to flow back into the chamber until the next time.

Premature ejaculation

Premature ejaculation is when the man ejaculates too early or even before penetration. It is defined as occurring within a minute of penetration. It is undoubtedly more common than we think because I am sure many men don't seek help. If this is something that you and your partner are happy with then that is fine, but if it is causing frustrations between you then it is important that you seek help.

What causes premature ejaculation?

Premature ejaculation is common in very young men and in the early stages of an exciting relationship. In this instance it usually improves spontaneously but if the problem persists there are a number of other possible causes including:

- psychological issues possibly dating back to early sexual experiences or related to anxiety;
- some prescription medicines;
- street drugs, such as cocaine and amphetamines;
- prostatitis (inflammation of the prostate);
- neurological diseases such as multiple sclerosis and conditions causing neuropathy.

What can I do to help myself?

If this is a new problem that has started with a new relationship the chances are it will settle without the need for you to do anything. You may find masturbating before sexual intercourse is helpful. Wearing thick condoms may reduce the sensation and delay ejaculation or you can ask your partner to go on top so that they can withdraw as you are about to orgasm and then resume when the sensation has settled. Alternatively your partner can masturbate you and if at the point you are about to orgasm they gently squeeze the head of the penis for 10–20 seconds the sensation should go away and you can continue. There are also devices that are held in your or your partner's palm that fit around the head of the penis and do a similar job.

Can my doctor help?

There are some anti-depressants that have been shown to delay ejaculation and there are also anaesthetic creams that reduce the sensation in the head of the penis, which may help. Your GP can also refer you for psychosexual counselling.

Retrograde ejaculation

Retrograde ejaculation is where semen enters the bladder instead of emerging from the penis at orgasm. The man will still experience an orgasm but may notice the urine is cloudy after having had sex. Retrograde ejaculation only really needs treating if it is causing problems with fertility. It can occur as a result of surgery to the prostate or bladder neck. Sometimes it is linked to other nerve problems such as multiple sclerosis or injury to the spinal cord and it can occur as a side effect of some medications used to treat high blood pressure, mood disorders or prostate enlargement. We can sometimes use drugs, which help to keep the bladder neck closed to help with retrograde ejaculation.

Priapism

A priapism is an erection that lasts several hours and causes pain. It happens when the blood flows into the penis to cause an erection but cannot flow out. It can be caused by vascular or neurological problems. It is more common in men who have a condition called sickle cell anaemia, which is an inherited condition associated with abnormal blood cells. It can occur as a result of using injections for ED and when using other drugs for high blood pressure, blood thinning or depression. It can also be seen in people using cocaine, ecstasy, crystal meth or cannabis. Much less commonly it can be seen in association with some cancers.

How is priapism treated?

Your doctor may need to aspirate the blood from your penis. He will use an local anaesthetic to numb the penis and then use a needle and syringe to relieve the erection. If this doesn't work, he can inject a drug, which is designed to squeeze the blood vessels in the penis and force the blood back out. Occasionally, we need to do an operation to relieve the priapism.

Balanitis

Balanitis is inflammation of the head (glans) of the penis. It is particularly common in young boys under 4 but it can affect men of any age. It is very uncommon in uncircumcized men. It causes the head of the penis to become red, inflamed and sore and it may also cause pain on passing urine.

What causes balanitis?

There are number of things that can predispose a man to developing balanitis.

- *Poor hygiene* Failure to clean under the foreskin can lead to build up of smegma (the cheesy substance which forms under the foreskin);
- *A tight foreskin* makes it difficult to retract the foreskin and therefore allows the build up of smegma;
- *Infection* Candida is the most common culprit here – the fungus that causes thrush in women – but balanitis can also be caused by chlamydia, gonorrhoea and herpes;
- *Allergy* Condoms, spermicides or chemicals on your hands can all cause an allergic reaction leading to balanitis;
- *Irritation* I have mentioned that poor hygiene can be responsible for balanitis but overzealous washing can also be to blame as it causes irritation.

What can I do to prevent balanitis?

Wash regularly with lukewarm water, remembering to clean under the foreskin. If you think you could be sensitive to soap, try using emollient cream instead. Dry your penis gently. Some of my patients have also told me that sitting in a bath with a few drops of tea tree oil is helpful.

Can my doctor help?

Your doctor may prescribe anti-fungal cream if he or she suspects thrush. He or she will treat any underlying STI and may prescribe a steroid cream to reduce the inflammation. If you have chronic or recurring balanitis it can lead to a condition called phimosis, where the foreskin cannot be properly retracted. In this instance your doctor will advise that you are referred for a circumcision.

Index